Caroline Chapman was born in India and spent her early childhood there. Educated at a 'bracing' school in North Yorkshire, she works as a picture-researcher and occasional writer. She is married to an explorer but does not accompany him on his major expeditions (apart from a three day camel ride in the Sahara), and has two children.

Dr. Caroline Lucas was brought up in London and Oxford. She trained at St. Mary's Medical School in London and did three years clinical training at Oxford University Medical School. After qualifying, Dr. Lucas spent two years in adult medicine at hospitals including the Radcliffe Infirmary and the Hammersmith Hospital, and four years in Paediatrics as Registrar at the Westminster Children's Hospital. She is at present working as Registrar in Radiotherapy/Oncology at the Royal Marsden Hospital.

The Pocket Holiday Doctor

Caroline Chapman
and
Dr. Caroline Lucas BM, B Ch.

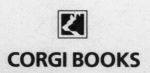

CORGI BOOKS

THE POCKET HOLIDAY DOCTOR
A CORGI BOOK 0 552 12195 9

First publication in Great Britain

PRINTING HISTORY
Corgi edition published 1983

This book is set in 10/11 Mallard

Corgi Books are published by
Transworld Publishers Ltd.,
Century House, 61–63 Uxbridge Road,
Ealing, London W5 5SA

Made and printed in Great Britain by
Cox & Wyman Ltd., Reading, Berks.

Acknowledgements

We would particularly like to thank Dr. Kenneth and Dr. Denise Hugh-Jones for their invaluable help and advice. We are also very grateful to Dr. Vanda Joss and Dr. Mira Leigh for reading the manuscript so carefully.

Special Note

We hope that you will find time to read this book *before* you go away on holiday. Some of the advice contained in it is only useful to you if you have acted on it before leaving. Some of it is advice on what to do in an emergency. For instance, you don't want to find yourself with a drowned person at your feet, and vital minutes ticking away whilst you look up Kiss-of-Life.

Contents

Introduction

'Getting away from it all' on holiday is wonderful, but there can be certain disadvantages: if you or one of your family becomes ill in any way, obtaining medical help can be very difficult and very expensive.

The idea for this book came to me last year in a remote part of southern Europe. My 10 year old daughter developed violent diarrhoea, vomiting and a high temperature. I suddenly realised that I really did not know what was the right thing to do to help her. The nearest telephone was half a mile away and was reputed to be highly temperamental. It was the middle of the night (of course) and even if the telephone had condescended to work, the nearest doctor was 10 miles away and there was absolutely no public transport. We would have had to beg, borrow or even steal a vehicle to get there. The journey would have been very uncomfortable for the child – although not actually harmful in this case.

Meanwhile, no less than four other strong-minded people were giving me contrary advice, nearly all of it wrong as it turned out. If I had possessed the basic knowledge as to how to treat severe diarrhoea and had known at what point a doctor had to be found, I would have been able to deal with the problem calmly and methodically.

This set of circumstances is by no means unusual. Surveys show that at least one in four people who go abroad on holiday have some sort of problem with their health, although the majority are only minor. Living in this country we take it for granted that there is a doctor or a casualty department on the end of a telephone (that works) day or night. It is not until you find yourself in the middle of a situation similar to mine that many of you will realise how ill-equipped you are to cope with it.

This book will advise you on what precautions to take before you go away on holiday and give you practical advice on what to do if you become ill when you are there. However, we can only give you *basic guidelines*: how you act upon them is up to you, your instinct, and your personal knowledge of whoever is ill.

AREAS COVERED BY THIS BOOK

Northern and Southern Europe

Turkey

North Africa

Middle East

South Africa

Australia and New Zealand

North America

USSR

Hong Kong

THIS BOOK DOES NOT DEAL WITH ANY OF THE FOLLOWING:

1. The Far East.
    Central and South America.
    The rest of Africa.

2. Although some of the advice contained in this book will be useful to 'over-landers' or those living rough, it is not specifically aimed at them. There are other excellent books on this subject.

3. Babies under about 2 years of age. You should consult your doctor about them.

4. Those who are going abroad for long periods. This is essentially a book for those going on holiday.

Note: Pregnant women and those who have an illness which requires special drugs must consult their doctor before going abroad.

1
THINGS TO THINK ABOUT BEFORE YOU GO

CLOTHES

If you are going somewhere hot, you must wear clothes, especially underclothes, made of *natural* fibre which can 'breathe', such as cotton. Try to wear light-coloured clothes without belts. Shoes should be as open as possible. Great big hats are not necessary, but a smaller hat with a brim is advisable, especially for small children, and they should be made to wear them whenever they are out in hot sun.

As your body acclimatises to the heat, your sweat glands begin to work more freely. Sweat can keep you cool but *only* if it is allowed to evaporate.

The glare of bright sun, especially off the surface of water, can be a problem. Sunglasses should be lightweight or polaroid.

TEETH

If you have not been to the dentist recently, now is your chance. Dentists abroad are difficult to find and very expensive.

TRAVEL SICKNESS

Children are notoriously travel sick but for over fives STUGERON, AVOMINE or MARZINE do help. If you are travelling by car, keep the windows open as much as possible and stop as often as you can for fresh air and a bit of a walk-about. Keep a child horizontal if it really feels miserable, take plenty of plastic bags and towels with you. It is obviously better not to travel on a full stomach.

If you are travelling by air, children in particular can suffer from painful ears due to the build-up of pressure. Chewing sweets or gum can help, especially during take-off and landing.

HEALTH INSURANCE

You will find the next section tedious reading but you *must* PERSEVERE – it is important. You would be very foolish to go on holiday abroad, especially if you have young children, without health insurance of any kind.

In general, the following information applies to you if you are a UK national resident in the UK. But if you are resident in the UK but a citizen of another country, it would be wise to contact the DHSS International Relations Division (for address see Chapter 2), who will tell you if your country has reciprocal health arrangements with the UK.

If you are going on holiday to one of the European Community (EC) countries (Belgium, Denmark, France, West Germany, Gibraltar, Greece, the Irish Republic, Italy, Luxembourg and Holland) then you can obtain urgent medical treatment free or at a reduced cost. This is a reciprocal arrangement between all EC countries.

However, this is all very complicated; EC countries differ considerably from each other as to what treatment is available. There are also (at time of publication) 17 other countries which have some sort of arrangement with the UK for urgent medical treatment. They are mainly in Northern Europe and Scandinavia but include the USSR, Australia and New Zealand.

But for more information about these countries and those in the EC, there is a Leaflet published by the Department of Health and Social Security (DHSS) which is recommended reading as it will tell you all you need to know.

It is Leaflet SA.30 'Medical Costs Abroad: What You Need To Know Before You Go!' and can be obtained from your local DHSS office or from; DHSS Leaflets Unit, PO Box 21, Stanmore, Middlesex HA7 1AY

On the back page of this Leaflet you will find a form CM.1 which you have to fill in, in order to get another Leaflet E111. You must have Leaflet E111 with you if you are on holiday in an EC country as you cannot obtain free or cheaper medical treatment without producing it. We strongly advise you to obtain one of these Leaflets, especially if you have young children, and to apply for it 1 to 6 months before you go away.

You haven't finished yet! With your Leaflet E111 you will be sent Leaflet SA.36 which tells you how to go about obtaining treatment, what sort of treatment you are entitled to, and how to claim for refunds. Therefore you must take this with you on holiday too.

But, when you have read the Leaflets, you may feel that the country you are going

19

to does not offer you sufficient free or cheap medical treatment – in which case you are *strongly advised* to take out some private insurance as well. (See following section.)

Believe it or not, all the above has been greatly simplified for the purpose of this book! But, as *you* will know which country (or countries) you are visiting, the whole thing becomes much easier as you can just look up the parts of the Leaflet which apply to you.

PRIVATE INSURANCE

If you are going to a country without reciprocal arrangements with the UK, or one that you feel does not give you adequate coverage, it would be *very unwise* not to take out private insurance. This can also cover the loss of your luggage. Most Travel Agents will arrange this for you, but it is up to you to ask for it. The premiums are not high and would be worth every penny if you were unlucky enough to fall ill.

CAR INSURANCE

If you are going abroad by car, the AA, RAC, and the Association of British Travel Agents have various schemes to help you. Some of these schemes include health insurance. You must ensure that you are covered for car breakdown and vehicle recovery and that you have a *green card* which is obligatory and enables you to drive abroad.

SUGGESTED MEDICAL KIT & CHECKLIST

Nearly all the following have been mentioned in the general text but we thought it would help to have a checklist:

Spare contact lenses and solution where applicable

Spare set of dentures

Supply of your prescribed contraceptive pills

Sea or air-sickness pills: AVOMINE: DRAMAMINE: STUGERON: (for over-five only)

Insect repellent: such as AUTAN

Insecticide: VAPONA or one of the MAFU range

Laxatives SENOKOT: MILPAR: MILK OF MAGNESIA

Water purifiers: STEROTABS: PURITABS

Rehydration salts: ORALYTE: DIOR-ALYTE (good for children)

Antiseptic creams such as SAVLON: CETAVLON

Antibiotic powder such as CICATRIN

Oral antihistamine pills such as PIRITON

Antihistamine creams such as ANTHI-SAN, CALADRYL

Anti-itching creams such as CALAMINE

For diarrhoea: LOMOTIL: DIOCALM: KAOLIN: KAOLIN & MORPHINE: ISOGEL: CODEINE-PHOSPHATE: For children KAOLIN MIXTURE

Anti-vomiting: STEMETIL: MAXOLON

For those who are very susceptible to the sun: UVISTAT

Toothache and mouth ulcers: BONJELA

Pain-killers such as PARACETAMOL (CALPOL for children) or ASPIRIN

For boils etc: MAGNESIUM SULPHATE paste

ELASTOPLAST in various sizes
Crepe bandage or TUBIGRIP

To prevent nappy rash: DRAPOLENE, ZINC & CASTOR OIL, VASOGEN

Sterile gauze dressings such as MELOLIN with surgical tape or roll of elastoplast to attach the dressing

Thermometer

Scissors

Sewing kit

Appropriate phrase book

DHSS Form E 111 see (HEALTH IN-SURANCE) pages 18–20.

2
IMMUNISATIONS—WHERE TO GO

This is a difficult subject because there are a number of immunisations which are ADVISABLE but not a MUST. You can obtain advice from your doctor, local infant welfare clinic, travel agent or the relevant country's Embassy. Embassies tend to play down the possibility of you catching a disease in their countries in order not to put you off going. On the other hand, you do not want to overdo the immunisations and set off on holiday feeling like a pincushion.

We have therefore given you the DHSS *recommended* immunisations to be on the safe side. However, what follows is only a guideline and if you are in any doubt, consult your doctor OR the following main centres:

1. The DHSS, Alexander Fleming House, Elephant & Castle, London SE1 6BY. Telephone: (01) 407 5522. Ask for the International Relations Division. They will give you advice only and not the immunisations themselves.

2. Your local DHSS office.

3. The Medical Department of British Airways, 75 Regent Street (Piccadilly

end), London W1. Telephone: (01) 439 9584. They will give you advice and do the immunisations for you at a cost of £2 each, upwards. No appointment is necessary but you can make one if you prefer. Opening hours: 8.30 am. – 4.30 pm. Monday to Friday.

4. The Vaccinating Centre, 53 Cumberland Place, London W1. Telephone: (01) 262 6456. Hours are 9 am. – 4.30 pm. Monday to Friday. No appointment necessary. £2.50 each, upwards.

5. Thomas Cook, 45 Berkeley Street, London W1. Telephone: (01) 499 9000. Open Monday to Friday and Saturday mornings. £3.00 each, upwards.

Note: Last minute immunisations can be done at:
Heathrow Airport, Terminal 3. Open 24 hours. Tel: (01) 759 5511
Gatwick Airport. Open 24 hours. Tel: (0293) 28822 Ext 3593.

COST

If you are going to a country where certain immunisations are obligatory (usually only Yellow Fever and Cholera), the National Health will do them free. But if the immunisations are just recommended, then you will have to pay for each one you have.

CERTIFICATES

Whoever has done the immunisations for you must also give you a signed certificate to prove that they have done so. You may

be required to show these to the
authorities of the country to which you are
going. If you do not live in London, the following is a list of regional immunisation
centres. Also included are two more
London centres, which provide special
advice on Yellow Fever, although this does
not come within the scope of this book.

Wales:

Welsh Office,
Cathays Park,
Cardiff CF1 3NQ,
Tel: (0222) 825111 Ext: 3395

Scotland:

Scottish Home & Health Dept.,
St. Andrew's House,
Edinburgh EH1 3DE
Tel: 031:5568501 Ext: 2438

For up to date information about vaccina-
tion requirements:
The Communicable Diseases (Scotland)
Unit,
Ruchill Hospital, Bilsand Drive,
Glasgow G20 9NB
Tel: 041 946 7120

England

Birmingham:

Immunisation Section,
1 Congreve Passage,
Birmingham B3 3DA
Tel: (021) 235 3428

Bristol:

Central Health Clinic,
GPO Box No. 201,

Tower Hill, Bristol.
Tel: (0272) 291010 Ext. 277

Lancaster:

Ashton Road Clinic,
Lancaster.
Tel: (0524) 2558

Leeds:

Leeds Area Health Authority (T)
Immunisation Centre,
Chapeltown Health Centre,
Spencer Place,
Leeds LS7 4 BB
Tel: (0532) 486351

Liverpool:

Area Health Authority Vaccination Clinic,
26 Hatton Garden,
Liverpool L3 2AW
Tel: 051 227 3911 Ext. 69

School of Tropical Medicine,
Pembroke Place,
Liverpool L3 5QA
Tel: (051) 227 3911

London:

Hospital for Tropical Diseases,
4 St. Pancras Way,
London NW1 OPE
Tel: (01) 387 4411 Ext. 136 or 137

Medical Department,
Unilever House,
Blackfriars, London EC4
Tel: (01) 822 6017

Manchester:

Basement Clinic,
Town Hall Extension,
Manchester M60 2JS
Tel: (061) 236 3377 Ext. 2554 & 2556

Truro:

Health Area Office,
The Leats,
Truro.
Tel: (0872) 2202

Northern Ireland:

Ballymena:

Yellow Fever Vaccination Centre,
51 Castle Street,
Ballymena.
Tel: (0266) 6324 or 2108

Belfast:

Dept. of Health & Social Services,
Lincoln Avenue Clinic,
Antrim Road,
Belfast BT14 6AZ.
Tel: (0232) 41771. Ext: 272

Omagh:

Western Health and Social Services
Board,
Yellow Fever Vaccination Centre,
The Health Centre,
Mountjoy Road,
Omagh.
Tel: (0662) 3521 Ext. 54

**NB. All addresses correct at time of going
to press.**

3
IMMUNISATIONS—WHICH TO HAVE

Many of the diseases covered in this book result from organisms (germs) themselves, or from the toxic substances that they produce. Immunisations provide a way of giving you the specific organism or toxin in a completely safe form so that you build up a resistance (become immune) to that particular disease. Thus, when you encounter the real disease (such as measles or tetanus) you should be sufficiently protected so that you will either not contract the disease at all, or at worst, only a very mild version of it.

REMEMBER that some of the immunisations need more than one dose for adequate protection to be achieved. So DO NOT leave it all to the last minute. Start thinking about it a few months before you go away.

Obviously, if an epidemic breaks out in the country to which you are going (such as the Cholera one in Spain in 1970) – then the risk is far greater and you would be very unwise not to have the relevant immunisation. But it is UP TO YOU to check.

BCG

This vaccine protects against Tuberculosis (TB). All British children are tested at school at about the age of 10 to see if they are immune or not. If they are not, they are then given the immunisation. TB is not a problem on holiday, only to those going abroad for long periods of time, like VSO workers. But it is a good idea to check that all members of the family are protected.

When the vaccine is given, a nodule appears after a few weeks and forms a small ulcer. But this will heal in 2–3 months and may leave a small scar. There might be a slight enlargement of the lymph glands under the arm but this is to be expected.

CHOLERA

This is a disease which can result from contaminated food and/or water, and has now spread to most countries except the Americas, Australia and New Zealand. You should seriously consider having this immunisation if you are going anywhere outside Northern Europe, or where sanitation is likely to be poor.

Also, as it is a disease which can occur in epidemic form, check that there is not one in the country to which you are going. In an epidemic you are not necessarily going to be protected even if you have had the immunisation.

The usual course consists of 2 injections at least two weeks apart and it does not become effective for 6 days. Protection lasts for 6 months.

INFECTIOUS HEPATITIS

This is an unpleasant disease which is also related to bad sanitation. So if you are going to a country where you have reason to suspect the sanitation will be poor, think seriously about this one. Consult your doctor or one of the other authorities to which we have referred.

There is an injection which (after a lot of controversy) the experts have agreed does give a good measure of protection. It is called GAMMA GLOBULIN and lasts for 3–6 months.

MALARIA

This is not only on the increase throughout the world but some strains are becoming resistant to existing drugs.

For the purposes of this book, the only areas (at the time of publication) in which you might contract malaria are those countries in North Africa which border the Mediterranean – including Egypt. The DHSS, however, *recommend* protection for Turkey, Mexico, South Africa and the Middle East.

There is no immunisation as such, but there are anti-malarial tablets which you take all the time you are abroad. Some are taken once a day and some once a week. Some you have to start taking two weeks before you go but all of them MUST continue to be taken for at least a month after you have returned.

There are a number of different drugs:

PALUDRINE   –   taken daily

CHLOROQUINE –   taken once a week
(there is a syrup for
children)

MALOPRIM   –   taken once a week

FANSIDAR   –   taken once a week (not recommended for pregnant women)

The Vaccinating Centre in London recommend the PALUDRINE and other authorities agree, because it is far less dangerous to forget to take one day's dose rather than one week's dose.

But you MUST obtain up to date advice on this from your doctor, or one of the addresses given previously, because different tablets are recommended for different countries. Also your doctor will know if any of them are unsuitable for you for some reason.

But, whichever one you use, you must devise a routine which suits your way of life so that it is *not* forgotten. The tablets are not on the National Health, but they are remarkably cheap to buy for what they are worth to you.

POLIOMYELITIS (POLIO)

This is an immunisation which seems to be completely forgotten by people going abroad on holiday. But if you are going to countries in North Africa in particular, or anywhere outside Northern Europe, North America, Australia and New Zealand, you must make sure that you and your family have full up to date immunisation.

Your children should have been immunised when babies and then had a booster at school-entry age and again at school-

31

leaving age. As an adult, you should have a booster at least once every five years, especially if you are going abroad.

REMEMBER that if you have never been immunised against polio then you must think ahead as it has to be given in 3 separate doses 6–8 weeks apart. It is taken in the form of 3 drops, usually on a sugar lump. If you have not had a booster for 10 years, you only need 2 doses, and if you have not had a booster for 5 years, you only need 1 dose.

RABIES

There is now a vaccine for this, but it is not usually recommended for those who are going abroad for a short period on holiday.

SMALLPOX

This has now been eradicated from the world. There has not been a case for 2 years – thanks to the work of the World Health Organisation. Immunisation is not needed for any of the areas covered by this book.

TETANUS

If you have never been immunised against it, this could be a good opportunity. Tetanus can be contracted anywhere, even at home, and at any time. Your children should have been immunised when babies when they were given the 'triple' vaccine (which consists of Diphtheria, Whooping-cough and Tetanus). A booster is given at school entry age and again at school leaving age. You should check when the last dose was given.

If you have not been immunised in the last 10 years, then you should have a booster. The course consists of three injections: the first and second should be given between 6 and 12 weeks apart and the third 6 months to a year later. Obviously, the third one causes a problem as it is so long after the first two. If you do not have time to have it before you go, which is highly likely, try and remember to have it sometime during the next year in order to complete the full course.

TYPHOID AND PARATYPHOID

This is yet another of the diseases which is spread by contaminated food and water. The old TAB vaccination has been discontinued as the A & B parts were found to be ineffective. The new one is Typhoid Monovalent which, incidentally, has fewer side effects although you can still have a very sore arm and possibly fever and feeling of nausea. The vaccination is about 50% effective.

The DHSS recommend it for all countries bordering the Mediterranean (including the Islands), Portugal, Bulgaria, Yugoslavia, the Canaries and South Africa. Of these, the North African countries are a MUST and Portugal and Spain should be seriously considered.

The ideal course is 2 injections with 4–12 weeks between them. This course will last you for 3 years. However, if you have left it too late for this, you can have 2 injections 10 days apart but you must then have a third injection in 9–12 months time. You will then be immunised for 3 years.

4

GENERAL ADVICE ON FOOD AND WATER

Some of the following advice you may find rather excessive. If you really took ALL these precautions, you might understandably feel that it is hardly worth the trouble of going to certain countries. But all we can do is to outline the various risks and how you can minimise them. Whether you follow the advice, and to what extent, *MUST* be up to you.

PRECAUTIONS

So many of the unpleasant things you can catch abroad are the result of food and water that have been contaminated by sewage. In other words, human or animal faeces have got into what you are eating or drinking, and this can happen in various ways. So, if you are on a self-catering holiday, or staying in an area where the sanitation is obviously poor, you must be especially careful.

DO NOT

Drink water that has not been boiled or purified in some way. (You can buy purifying tablets at the chemist; see Chapter 1)
    Eat locally made ice-cream.

Use ice cubes in your drinks as these tend to be made of local water.

Eat food which has been standing around, i.e. on display in a restaurant, particularly if there are a *lot of flies about*.

Eat food which has been re-heated. This is a difficult one because you can only be really sure if you are on a self-catering holiday.

Swim in obviously contaminated water.

Eat underdone meat or fish.

Eat shell-fish and tinned meat as they are also rather suspect, but you must just use your common sense about these.

DO

Wash fresh fruit, vegetables and salad ingredients in water that has been sterilised, peel, where possible. Don't leave it standing around uncovered.

Always wash your hands after you have been to the lavatory – children in particular find this one hard to remember.

Boil milk – or drink sterilised milk. Use sterilised cream if possible.

5
EFFECTS OF SUN AND HEAT

Although most people know how easily the sun can burn, it is astonishing how many holiday-makers choose to ignore this fact. Here are some guidelines for sunbathing.

1. Start your sunbathing very slowly; 15–30 minutes only for the first day and then increase this gradually. This will seem maddeningly slow to those who have under two weeks abroad. For those who have been exposed to strong sun before and know how their skin reacts, you can adjust this programme accordingly.

2. Remember that the effects of the sun do not appear immediately – usually not until the evening. So just because you have hardly changed colour at the time, this does not mean that the sun has not burned you.

3. You can become sunburnt even when there is a haze over the sun, or cloud or even fog ... the sun's rays can penetrate all these.

4. A breeze will speed up the process, so beware. Sitting in an open moving boat

is one of the most hazardous of all. The breeze keeps your skin nice and cool, but do not be fooled by this. Even veteran sunbathers can be caught this way.

5. Sun reflected off water has added power – as you will notice when you try and look at it. The glare is far greater.

6. Avoid the mid-day sun. This is when it is strongest.

7. Wash the salt off your skin when you have finished swimming for the day, or each time you come out of the sea if there is a shower handy.

Note: If you have especially sensitive skin, i.e. you have red hair, very fair hair and blue eyes, very fair skin or freckles, take particular care. There is a barrier cream called UVISTAT which will give you considerable protection, but you will not get a sun tan when using it.

SUN TAN LOTIONS

Use a *good* sun-tan lotion liberally – although they are very expensive. Look for the ones which have a SPF (sun protection factor) number on them, or a formula number. These range from 1 – 10 (or 15). *The higher the number the greater the protection*, and naturally, the slower you will tan. You may want to take a high number for the beginning of the holiday and a low number for when your skin has become less sensitive and you want to speed up the tanning process.

Remember that after a long swim, you should reapply the lotion. There are a few lotions which are water-resistant. Some people find they are sensitive to certain lotions so try and find which one suits your skin.

There are now a number of good sun tan lotions made principally from natural ingredients. They seem to be cheaper than the big brand names and can be found in most health food shops.

SUNBURN

If areas of your skin have become hot, red and sore to the touch, try the following:

Have a cool shower or bath and dab yourself dry.

Apply CALAMINE liberally. In Turkey we spread the local natural yoghurt on our sunburn which was wonderfully cooling.

If the skin has become swollen, very red and starts to blister, you must be careful not to let it become infected. Keep the area clean and dry and try to resist peeling the blisters off before they are ready. You must keep out of the direct sun until your skin has healed. An antihistamine tablet will help ease the irritation. Vitamin E oil spread over the burnt area is also a help – you will have to pierce the capsules to get at the oil.

We stupidly lay for 2 hours under a hazy sun last year in Sardinia and were very burnt. A passing traveller gave us this following tip: eat sliced skinned tomatoes with a sprinkle of salt. We tried it and it was very helpful, but don't give this

38

to very young children.

If the sunburn is *really* bad, see a doctor.

HEAT EXHAUSTION

This is usually caused by people coming suddenly from a cool climate into a very hot one – and doing too much before they are properly acclimatized.

Symptons and Signs:

>   Sweating
>   Feeling cold and clammy
>   No fever but possibly feeling of weakness and vertigo
>   Possible fainting
>   Pulse and breathing become rapid

Treatment:

Lie the person down in a cool room and give them cold water to drink. If they have been sick or had diarrhoea or muscular cramps, add a level teaspoon of salt to each pint (approx. ½ litre or 2½ teacups) of water they drink. If they feel better after a while, there is no need to get a doctor. But this state can sometimes deteriorate and become HEAT STROKE.

HEAT STROKE

This is very serious. It can be preceded by Heat Exhaustion as above, or it may come on suddenly. However, a person is unlikely to suffer from this condition unless they are in a *very* hot climate, or they have a chronic disease (such as diabetes or heart trouble) or they are elderly.

Heat stroke is basically caused by the failure of the body's thermostat, which means that you *cannot* sweat adequately. Therefore, all the heat is bottled up in the body, the temperature goes up high (sometimes to 104°F/40°C or more). The person feels dizzy, faint and may lose consciousness. The skin will be hot, dry and red.

GET MEDICAL HELP IMMEDIATELY

In the meantime, the most effective treatment is to immerse the patient in a tepid bath. This may sound very drastic, but you MUST get their temperature down quickly, and this is the quickest way. If there is no bath, another method is to strip the patient and wrap him in a wet, cold sheet for a short time. Keep it wet and cold until the temperature comes down to not less than 101°F (38°C). Then keep sponging him with tepid water to allow the sweat to evaporate in order to keep the temperature down. This applies to the bath method as well – as soon as the fever is down to 101°F (38°C) remove the patient to a cool room.

If the temperature begins to go up again, repeat the bath or sheet process until professional help arrives. Massage the skin as well, as this aids the flow of cooler blood around the body. Remember to persuade the patient to drink lots of fluid.

6
DIARRHOEA

This can be quite a problem on holiday, particularly if you have young children. You can become quite worried and everyone is inclined to give you contrary advice as to what to do. But REMEMBER that if you follow certain simple rules and procedures, it can usually be dealt with quite easily by you. Diarrhoea should not last for more than 1–3 days, and should never have blood in it, (see page 45)

Causes:

There are many, but the following are the most common: change of diet; unhygienic food preparation; bad sanitation; the use of a lot of olive oil which can act as a laxative; the local wine – and so on. Don't spend time trying to pin down where you got it from because nine times out of ten you will be wrong.

Symptoms:

Don't worry if your trips to the lavatory are a little more frequent and the stools looser during the first week abroad. What IS important is if you have constant very loose or watery stools. These may be accompanied by nausea or vomiting or sharp cramps in the abdomen which come and go. Occasionally, it may be accompanied by a temperature (see FEVER page 50)

Prevention:

We do not advise taking preventative medicines in any situation. If you take precautions as outlined earlier, all should be well.

However, if you are on a short business trip for instance, and it is imperative that you do not run into problems of an upset stomach, research has suggested that tablets called STREPTOTRIAD, taken twice a day for up to a maximum of four weeks, can lessen your chances of developing diarrhoea. It is only available on a doctor's prescription and should be started the day that you travel.

FOR SOME PRECAUTIONS ONCE YOU ARE ABROAD SEE 'GENERAL ADVICE ON FOOD AND WATER' in Chapter 4

Treatment (once you have diarrhoea):

You can take any of the following tablets, but remember that they only relieve the symptoms, they do NOT cure the diarrhoea. In fact, some authorities maintain that they just act as a 'plug'. They can also mask the symptoms of something more serious:-

LOMOTIL: DIOCALM: KAOLIN: KAOLIN & MORPHINE: IMODIUM: CODEINE-PHOSPHATE (also good as a pain-killer). KAOLIN MIXTURE should be safe for children but you should obtain advice on dosage before going abroad.

42

The MOST IMPORTANT thing to remember is that diarrhoea causes a considerable loss of fluid, leading to dehydration, which MUST be replaced, so you must drink as much as possible. (see DEHYDRATION page 49)

SAFE TO DRINK ARE (clear fluids)

Weak tea
Rice water (water from boiled rice)
Fizzy drinks which have gone flat
Liquidised orange, banana and added glucose
Chicken, meat, egg or bean broth
The best of all, particularly for children is a REHYDRATION DRINK (see DEHYDRATION page 49)

DO NOT DRINK

Strong coffee
Alcohol
Milk
Unpurified water (if possible)

FOOD

When the patient starts to improve, give diluted *boiled* milk in gradually increasing strengths, until the patient is able to tolerate milk at full strength. This may take 36–72 hours. Then you should start trying to get some food down, in small quantities, as soon as the patient feels up to it, even if it doesn't appear to be helping much at first.

SAFE TO EAT

Bread
Ripe bananas
Rice (boiled)
Raw apple, finely grated and very ripe
(good for children)
Potatoes
Dry biscuits (e.g. crackers)
Well-cooked chicken, fish or meat
Pulses, such as lentils (well-cooked and
mashed)

DO NOT EAT

Any greasy foods or those cooked in fat
and oil
Highly seasoned foods, although Indian
Dal is excellent as it is made from lentils
Unpeeled fruit and tomatoes

Antibiotics

These are not advisable, except when prescribed by a doctor. They may make the
situation worse – some antibiotics *cause*
diarrhoea! Or you may be hiding the symptoms of something else (see ANTIBIOTICS
page 87.)

Temperature/fever

If the diarrhoea is accompanied by a
temperature, you can take something to
help bring the temperature down.
PARACETAMOL is the best for children,
but limit it to the prescribed four-hourly
dose.
  The mistake so many anxious mothers
make is to keep the child with a temperature warm and covered up. Your aim is to

cool the child down. So don't cover him up. Keep the room as cool as possible. You can sponge him down with *tepid* water and give him cold drinks. (For more detailed information see FEVER page 50)

The following are all situations when you *MUST GET A DOCTOR*:

1. a) If the child is less than 2 years old and has had bad diarrhoea for 12–24 hours.
    b) For children between 2 years and 10 years (if they are otherwise well): if they have had moderate diarrhoea (5 stools a day) for more than *3 days*: OR if the diarrhoea is severe (10 stools a day) then they must see a doctor after 2 days.
    c) For children over 10 (if they are otherwise well): if they have had moderate diarrhoea for 5 days, or if the diarrhoea is severe, they must see a doctor after 3 days.

2. If there is any blood, or blood and mucus, in the stools.

3. Persistent abdominal pain for more than 6 hours.

4. If a child has a dry tongue or looks drowsy or vacant, or is not passing urine as much as usual, i.e. has dry nappies for more than 6 hours (in other words, he is becoming DEHYDRATED. See page 49)

5. Vomiting. i.e. if you feel nothing is staying down at all OR if drink

is being refused.

6.   If there are any additional symptoms, a rash for instance.

7.   If you already had some other medical condition before going abroad and you then develop diarrhoea, the whole situation must be treated more seriously.

8.   If you know that diseases such as CHOLERA and TYPHOID are in the area, then obviously you must be much more on your guard.

9.   If a child less than 5 years old has a temperature of 101°F (38°C) for more than 24 hours.

DYSENTERY

This is diarrhoea with blood and is highly endemic in North Africa, Turkey and the Middle East. There are two types, Amoebic and Bacillary, the latter being the most common. They are both spread by contaminated food and water.

Amoebic Dysentery

Symptoms

Starts gradually with 3 or 4 loose stools a day increasing to about 12 a day
    These become semi-liquid and smell bad
    They contain blood and mucus
    Stomach pains can be acute
    Seldom accompanied by fever

Bacillary Dysentery

Symptoms:

Severe diarrhoea which comes on suddenly
Temperature rising to 100–102°F or 38–39°C
Nausea but not necessarily vomiting
You may have to 'go' 15–30 times a day
Blood and mucus in the stools
Sharp stomach cramps and painful straining

Treatment for both:

You MUST be treated by a doctor for these. He will investigate which one you have, which is VITAL as they are treated in different ways. Amoebic dysentery is treated with a specific drug and must be cleared up as soon as possible as it can lead to complications with the liver.

Treatment for Bacillary dysentery is also specific and must be prescribed by a doctor.

7

ABDOMINAL PAIN, DEHYDRATION, FEVER, VOMITING

ABDOMINAL PAIN

One of the commonest causes of this abroad is food poisoning, but this should only last for 1–3 days. The pain can be sharp and tends to come and go. (For detailed information see DIARRHOEA, Chapter 6 and STAPHYLOCOCCUS page 69.)

If you get constant *discomfort* or pain, then you must find a doctor. If it is ignored, there is a possibility that the bowel may be inflamed and the situation can then become much more serious. As pain killers will mask the symptoms, try not to take any until the doctor has seen the patient.

The very young and the elderly sometimes find it difficult to explain exactly where the pain is. But if they complain of pain which is *constant*, get a doctor.

APPENDICITIS

This is a common surgical emergency, especially in the younger age group. The pain often begins in the upper stomach area and then moves to the right side of the stomach in the lower half – but this is not always the case (just to make life difficult). The pain may be accompanied by nausea, vomiting and a temperature. (Any persistent pain for more than 6 hours is suspicious until proved otherwise).

I think a lot of people have a fear of not diagnosing Appendicitis in time, or of being miles from anywhere when they get it. But I know two people who both got it on top of a mountain, one in South America and one in Greenland, and they both lived to tell the tale – although they may have been lucky.

DEHYDRATION

In a normal situation there is a *balance* between the fluids that the body takes in and the amount that you get rid of in the urine, from the bowel, and when you sweat. If the loss of fluid *exceeds* the intake, such as in diarrhoea and vomiting, the patient can become dehydrated. In some cases this can happen very quickly indeed – (see CHOLERA page 54.) But if it happens to the very young or very old, it is always serious.

Remember that in a hot climate or if the patient has a fever, the loss of fluids will be greater because of the sweating, For any illness that includes diarrhoea and/or vomiting, give the patient the following drink:

REHYDRATION DRINK (not suitable for those under 2 years old)

To one litre of water (2½ cups) – preferably boiled (but not boiling) – add two level tablespoons of sugar or honey and enough salt to just make it taste (¾ small level teaspoon but *no more*). If you are using pints, then it would be one small (2.5gm) level teaspoon of salt to two pints.

You can add ½ cup of orange juice or a little mashed ripe banana, which not only helps physically but makes it taste better.

Give this drink in small sips at 5–10 minute intervals. Even if the person is being sick, enough of the drink may stay down to do some good, but you MUST persevere.

Note: You can buy sachets of REHYDRATION SALTS which you dilute with water. There are also sachets which are especially good for babies called DIORYLATE, which you dilute strictly as directed. These can both be obtained from chemists in the UK.

Amounts of the drink to give:

These vary according to the severity of the diarrhoea. To whatever the person *normally* drinks in a day (and this of course increases in a hot climate) must be added what you estimate they have lost in the diarrhoea and/or vomiting. Err on the side of too much liquid rather than too little.

The *first* symptoms of dehydration include a dry tongue and not passing urine so frequently – dry nappies for example, when you would normally expect to be changing them. In this situation, *you must get a doctor*, since these signs may progress to lethargy prior to more serious complications.

FEVER

When an adult has a fever, it is uncomfortable but not dangerous in itself. When a child (especially below the age of 6 years) has a fever, it may cause problems and you must persevere to lower the temperature and to prevent it from rising again. Obviously there must be a cause for the fever and this should be found.

Method for lowering the temperature:

Remove the child's clothes and do all you can to keep him cool. Sponge him down with cool flannels or cloths that have been soaked in cool water, and encourage him to take cold drinks. Although it sounds an awful thing to do to a sick child, it may be necessary to sit the child in a tepid bath to lower the temperature.

In addition to these measures, give PARCETAMOL or CALPOL, according to the instructions on the bottle.

The reasoning behind all these measures is that some young children are prone to 'febrile convulsions' or 'fits' which can be largely prevented if care is taken to lower the temperature and to keep it down. It is important to realise that the convulsion does not occur necessarily at the height of the temperature but as it is rising.

If a child does have a funny turn, you must see a doctor immediately. If you have to take him to the doctor, remember NOT to wrap him up as he will only overheat even more.

TEMPERATURE GUIDE

C°	F°	
37	98.4	normal
38–39	99–102	there is some fever
39–42	102–108	high to very high fever

Over 40°C or 104°F the fever is getting dangerously high and you MUST find a doctor.

VOMITING

This will most commonly be associated with an upset stomach and diarrhoea. Unless you have any of the following symptoms, just take it easy and drink clear fluids until you feel able to eat again. (For general advice on this see DIARRHOEA, Chapter 6.)

Get a doctor in the following circumstances:

If it continues for more than 12 hours or if there is no obvious cause

If there is an associated headache (see MENINGITIS page 91.)

If there has been a head injury

If there is blood or bile in the vomit

If the patient is ill in any other way, i.e. has a temperature

If the patient is a young child and the vomiting is obviously associated with the diarrhoea

If the patient has persistent pain in the stomach for more than 6 hours.

8
INTRODUCTION TO INFECTIOUS DISEASES

Many of the infectious diseases covered in
this book – i.e. Infectious Hepatitis,
Typhoid, Polio – as you will see, start with
a variety of 'flu-like' symptoms of which
you would normally not take much notice.
It is very unlikely that you will become ill
with any of these diseases if you are only
on a short holiday. However, if you develop
'flu-like' symptoms when you return from
abroad, and they persist for more than 2 or
3 days, consult your doctor and remember
to tell him where you have been.

BRUCELLOSIS (There is no immunisation
for this)

This is caught from animals, mainly cattle,
sheep, goats and pigs – either from the
milk or from direct contact with an
infected animal. So, avoid drinking
unboiled milk if possible. In areas where
you know this disease exists, it would be
wise to avoid the local cheese as it may
have been made from unboiled milk.

    The incubation period may be from a
few days to a few weeks, so the chances
are that you will be back in this country
before it develops.

Symptoms:

> Fever and headache (see FEVER, HEADACHE, etc. page 50.)
>> Tiredness
>> Pains in the joints
>> Sweating

Treatment:

If you feel generally unwell and have these symptoms for more than 1–2 days, a doctor should be contacted. These symptoms are all very non-specific but if you stick to the rules for FEVER AND HEADACHE, you should be alright. But, if you are *in any doubt at all*, find a doctor.

CHOLERA

Results from contaminated food and water. This can be very dangerous as it can come on very suddenly, and can lead to dehydration very quickly.

Symptoms:

> Very severe diarrhoea which starts as normal watery stools but then these become completely watery, possibly with mucus (slime) in them – referred to as 'rice-water stools'.

Vomiting:

> Rapid and severe dehydration which can be accompanied by headache.

FEVER: see Dehydration chapter 7

> At the first signs of the diarrhoea becoming completely watery, you should contact the doctor *immediately* – especially if there is Cholera in the area.

Treatment:

Hopefully, you will be on your way to hospital, but if there is any delay getting there, it is VITAL to maintain hydration. (See DEHYDRATION Chapter 7.) You MUST continue to drink, even if it is only in small sips. A litre (1 ¾ pints) or more, every four hours. If you normally have no medical problems (i.e. kidney or heart disease) you CANNOT drink too much in these circumstances.

INFECTIOUS HEPATITIS

Results from contaminated food and water. Incubation period is 15 to 50 days (usually about 25) and so you must report to a doctor when you return if you have the following:

Symptoms:

Fever
Marked loss of appetite and energy
Nausea
Abdominal pains
Skin and whites of the eyes turn yellow after a few days.
Urine turns deep orange or the colour of weak tea
Stools turn colourless.

Treatment:

Although there is no specific medicine for this disease, get medical help. Do not smoke, although you probably won't feel like it, and rest as much as possible.

Do not drink alcohol at the time, and for at least 6 months afterwards.

Drink as much of the REHYDRATION DRINK (see page 49) as possible, or orange juice or any of those drinks under DIARRHOEA page 41. When you feel like eating again, have fat free foods and fruit until you are back to normal.

Note: As this is very infectious, take the same precautions as under TYPHOID page 61.

MALARIA

This is caused by a special type of mosquito which injects the infection into the blood when it bites you. There are four main types and one of the four is more likely to be fatal than the others. As the incubation period can be anything from 10–28 days, report any fever which occurs as soon as you return from an area where Malaria is endemic.

Precautions:

As the malaria-carrying mosquitoes usually bite when it is dusk or dark, always cover yourself up as much as possible at this time.

Use insect sprays in the room at night. (see page 71)

Use slow-burning mosquito coils near your bed at night – these can usually be bought locally.

Cover any exposed skin liberally with insect repellent if you go out at night. (see page 71)

Hopefully, if you are in an area where Malaria is rife, your accommodation will provide you with mosquito nets or have windows which are covered in wire mesh.

Symptoms:

>Starts with chills and shivering
>Often headache
>Often nausea and vomiting
>High temperature, often rising to 40°C (104°F) or more.

Note: You MUST get a doctor now. The next stage is possibly delirium. Don't forget that Malaria can be a dangerous disease.

After several hours the patient will start to sweat and the temperature usually begins to go down.

Treatment:

The doctor will treat you with the appropriate medicine, which may have to be administered intravenously.

POLIO

This disease is world-wide but epidemics are limited to a small number of areas, usually where sanitation is poor. The incubation period is 3–35 days. The virus is carried in the stools.

Symptoms:

>Headache
>Sore throat
>Fever
>Diarrhoea and vomiting (see DIARRHOEA page 41.)
>Abdominal pain (see page 48.)
>Sore and aching muscles followed by paralysis

Treatment:

You MUST check these symptoms against those given in DIARRHOEA and

ABDOMINAL PAIN. If you are in *any* *doubt* at all, and particularly if you have heard of polio being in the area, you MUST find a doctor. This is a very serious illness as I am sure you know, and although there is no specific treatment, you must be in hospital and under constant medical supervision.

Keep the patient in bed and prevent him from using his muscles.

If there is any delay in getting to hospital, give the patient ASPIRIN to help the pain and bring down the temperature if there is one.

If there is *no fever*, you can put hot towels on the sore muscles to help ease the discomfort.

Note: Keep everyone else away from the patient and the person who is doing the nursing should wash his hands very thoroughly after touching him.

RABIES

This is a horrible illness but you would be very unlucky if you contracted it on holiday if you take precautions, especially in the areas dealt with by this book.

Before going to a country where it is possible to catch Rabies, one tends to imagine that rabid dogs, foaming at the mouth, will come staggering round every corner. When you actually get there, the danger is that you seem to forget about them altogether.

The Rabies virus is in the saliva of the infected animal, so even if you are licked by a rabid dog or cat or some rodents and bats and you have any 'broken skin' (i.e. a scratch or a graze) the infection can enter that way. Dogs are the most common carriers, so STOP your children from approaching strange dogs abroad. In fact, it should be assumed that any animal abroad may have rabies.

Signs of Rabies in an ANIMAL:

Behaves in a restless, agitated way
Possibly trembling or growling
Possibly foaming at the mouth, unable to drink
Possibly partial paralysis will have set in and the dog's hind legs may keep giving way

If you get bitten or licked by a dog suspected of being Rabid:

Immediately flush out the wound with a great deal of soapy water, detergent or alcohol – for at least 5 minutes. Or run it under the tap. But whatever you do, do it thoroughly. Get someone to locate the owner of the dog as soon as possible, see later.

THEN GET TO A DOCTOR OR HOSPITAL AT ONCE

It depends where in the body you have been bitten as to how long the period of incubation is – but about 30 days is the minimum period. It is more serious with large bites – and with children. The doctor or hospital will administer treatment as appropriate and the course may continue for several days. But this MUST be done as Rabies nearly always kills unless the appropriate treatment is given.

Signs of Rabies in HUMANS:

Fever, loss of appetite, headache, nausea, sore throat, sensitivity around the wound, muscular aches, sometimes a fear of water develops and then paralysis.

Note: You MUST try and find the owner of the animal and establish if it has been immunised against rabies. Ask to see the certificates to prove it. The owner should keep the animal shut up for 7–10 days. If it is still alive by the end of the period, then it could NOT have had rabies.

You must inform the local police.

TETANUS

This occurs when the organism, which is present in the soil or in human and animal stools, has contact with an open wound. This can be a hazard for superficial wounds if you are in an area with Tetanus, but you must especially TAKE GREAT CARE with a deep wound.

Typical examples of injuries which can become infected include barbed wire, nails, fish hooks, etc. Or if you get a deep burn, or if you break a bone badly and the skin is also 'broken'.

You *should have been immunised*, but even if you have and have also had a booster within the last 10 years (see IMMUNISATIONS, Chapter 3) you MUST clean the wound thoroughly (see CUTS, BREAKS, ETC page 65–66) and get to a doctor. He may decide to give you an additional booster and antibiotics.

Symptoms:

Hopefully, these will not start before you get to hospital, but they may include spasms near the site of the wound, rigid muscles, the jaw becomes stiff and won't open properly (hence one of the other names for it – LOCKJAW) and convulsions. If you should be unlucky enough to have one of the family develop these symptoms out of hospital, then move the patient as little as possible, avoid bright lights and get to a hospital immediately.

TUBERCULOSIS (TB or Consumption)

This disease comes from inhaling the infectious material and may also occur from drinking infected milk. It principally affects the lungs. This should not be a problem on holiday but see under IMMUNISATION page 23 for more information.

The symptoms include a chronic cough, generally being unwell with loss of weight and sweating, but there are *many* other possible symptoms, so don't try to diagnose yourself.

TYPHOID AND PARATYPHOID

Also results from contaminated food and water. This is another potentially very dangerous disease but comes on less suddenly than Cholera. The incubation period is 10–14 days so if you feel unwell and have a fever on your return home, contact your doctor immediately.

Symptoms:

During First Week
General feeling of being unwell

Headache and sore throat – see HEADACHE page 90.
Dry cough
Possible constipation or diarrhoea
Vomiting
Abdominal pains

Note: If there is Typhoid in the area and you now begin to get a fever, you MUST find a doctor immediately. The temperature will go up a little each day until it reaches 40°C (104°F) or more. Also, if you have had the above symptoms for more than three days, you must get a doctor.

During Second Week (or sooner)
Start of diarrhoea
High fever, pulse relatively slow
Trembling and delirium
Red spots sometimes appear on the tummy
Weight loss and dehydration

Treatment:

If you have to wait for medical help, you should drink the REHYDRATION Drink (see page 49.)

Lower the fever with cool, wet cloths or sponging (see FEVER page 50.) In hospital you will probably be treated with antibiotics or given fluids intravenously by means of a drip.

Note: As this is a VERY infectious disease and the germs are carried in the stools, the persons dealing with the patient MUST be careful to wash his hands thoroughly and repeatedly.

9

BURNS, CUTS, BREAKS AND OTHER MINOR DISASTERS

BOILS/ABSCESSES

If these are limited to a specific area of the body and the person is otherwise completely well, try and remove the pus from the boil.

Use very hot, moist, clean pads on top of the area. Magnesium Sulphate paste may be used under the dressing. As soon as the pad has cooled down, repeat the process. It is important that the pus comes out.

Do NOT squeeze the boil since this may spread the infection. When the boil has discharged, leave it uncovered if possible and allow it to drain.

If the redness begins to spread around the boil, or the glands become swollen, or the person seems unwell in any other way, get a doctor. He may need to have antibiotics and special dressings on the boil.

BURNS AND SCALDS

Minor: Immerse the burn immediately in cold water (not seawater) and keep it there for about 10 minutes. Take ASPIRIN if necessary (but it shouldn't be). This is *all* you need to do.

Not so Minor: (i.e. causes blisters). *Don't* prick the blisters. *Don't* smear on grease,

63

such as butter, and *don't* use cotton wool. Just cover the burn with a sterile dressing and bandage lightly.

Don't forget that you are in strange surroundings and whereas your child will have been warned against touching things on the stove at home, he may not associate these warnings with the new place.

If a child has a burn, it is obviously more serious and medical advice should be sought, sooner rather than later.

Major Burns: GO TO THE DOCTOR

CONJUNCTIVITIS

The eye becomes sticky with pus and difficult to open in the mornings. The white of the eye may be a bit red. If these symptoms continue for a day without clearing up at all, you may need antibiotic drops, so try and find a doctor.

As with other problems in young children, take this more seriously and find a doctor. Remember, this is very infectious so wash your hands thoroughly after touching the eyes.

Also make sure that there is not a foreign body in the eye, i.e. a hair, grit etc., and if so remove it. Take a very clean handkerchief and with the corner, gently remove the object. You may have to bend back the upper eye-lid completely to get at a foreign body underneath, but this will easily right itself when the person blinks. If you continue to have discomfort, get medical advice.

CUTS AND WOUNDS

Small cuts: The important point is to *clean* it and *keep* it clean. Wash it really well, preferably with boiled water with a little salt in it, or soap. Make sure there are no 'foreign bodies' left in it, such as grit, splinters and especially glass. Do not cover it with plaster as this will stop the air getting in and the pus (if there is any) getting out. You can put on an antiseptic cream such as SAVLON or CETAVLON, or you can apply GENTIAN VIOLET or MERCURICHROME.

Although seawater contains both salt and iodine, you will find that if you are swimming a lot, your cuts will take a long time to heal. This is because they never get a chance to dry out properly.

Splinters: These will have to be removed or the area may go septic. Sterilise a sewing needle by passing it through a flame several times. Allow it to cool (although don't test it by touching it) and then remove the splinter.

Large Wounds

Wash very throughly with boiled water and salt, or soap, until absolutely clean – you can actually pour the boiled water (not boiling) into the wound. If the cut is gaping open, try and close the sides together and then apply a sterile gauze dressing. Stick this down with some zinc-oxide tape until you can get to a doctor and have it stitched.

If the wound is bleeding badly, put a clean pad over it and press down firmly and keep pressing until the bleeding stops, but make sure foreign bodies are removed first. (See FOREIGN BODIES Page 66)

If it won't stop, then put on a tourniquet but *only until you can get a doctor*. Using a wide cloth or belt (not thin string or anything similar) tie it tightly around the limb, as close to the wound as possible, and between it and the rest of the body.

But you must only do this for a very short time as you could stop the circulation altogether. Loosen the tourniquet every half hour to see if the bleeding has stopped. (Obviously if the wound is somewhere like the neck or scalp, only apply pressure over the wound itself).

Keep the limb as high as possible i.e. above the level of the chest. Then get to a doctor for stitches.

Note: If the wound is deep, be VERY CAREFUL. (See TETANUS Chapter 8). If, after a few days, the wound is refusing to heal or there is redness of the skin around it, or the person is unwell and/or has a fever, get medical help.

FOREIGN BODIES

All foreign bodies, wherever they are, *must be removed*. Children frequently stuff things in their ears, up their noses, or any available orifice, and these must be *gently* removed. More seriously, an object such as a fish bone may get stuck in the gullet (the passage between the mouth and the stomach) or an object may be inhaled (see CHOKING page 80.)

An object in the eye:

If the object is something like grit or an eyelash then try to remove it with the corner of a clean handkerchief. It is easy to look under the lower eyelid, and the upper eyelid may be bent back to look underneath. If you cannot remove the object, go to a hospital.

If the object cannot be found or is lying in the surface of the eyeball, then cover the eye with a clean dressing and go to a hospital (see CONJUNCTIVITIS.)

Object in Ears and Nose:

Objects in the nose can normally be dislodged by giving it a good blow. Do not attempt to remove it if there is any chance of pushing it further up the nose. Get medical help.

If an object is in the ear and cannot be easily removed without pushing it further down the ear canal, then get medical help.

Swallowed Objects:

If the object was smooth and small, i.e. coins or pebbles, then it will probably appear in the stools a few days later without causing further problems.

If it has lodged in the back of the throat, it may be enough to make the person cough by slapping him on the back.

If the object is sharp, i.e. a chicken or fish bone, then you must get medical help.

Inhaled Objects:

(see CHOKING page 80.)

FRACTURES

You may be unlucky enough to break a bone, or crack it (a hair-line fracture). In either event, the limb must be set in plaster by an expert.

Always make sure that the potentially more dangerous injuries, such as bleeding or breathing difficulties, have been dealt with first.

Leg Fracture:

Your aim is to keep the leg COMPLETELY still in order to minimise movement of the bones across the site of the fracture. While you are waiting for medical help, keep the patient quiet and do not move him. Do NOT give him anything to eat or drink.

If you think that medical help may take a long time to come, you can make a splint with two slabs of wood on either side of the broken limb with a scarf or tie or belt tied around the limb, keeping the slabs in position.

Arm Fracture:

Immobilise the patient's arm by putting it in a sling i.e. a tie or belt tied around the back of the neck.

But, if the arm appears to be broken at the elbow, the arm must be kept straight.

If the patient seems to be relatively well, don't wait for medical help but take him to the nearest hospital.

NOSEBLEEDS

Sit upright and pinch the nose firmly for 10 minutes at least. If it is a young child, you will have to do it for him. Lying down just means that all the blood goes down the back of the throat, which children hate, and anyway it doesn't help. If the patient feels faint, then they will have to either sit on a chair with the head between the knees, or lie on the floor.

I was always having nosebleeds as a child and remember being made to spend long periods lying on the floor with a bunch of keys (for some odd reason) down the back of my neck, which is useless.

When the bleeding has stopped, try and stop the child touching or blowing its nose for as long as possible, although it is a great temptation to do so. Obviously, if the bleeding will not stop, or keeps occurring, consult a doctor.

STAPHYLOCOCCUS

This is a bacterium ('staph') which lives in the nose and on the skin and commonly causes boils, styes, spots etc. It is also one of the commonest causes of infected wounds (see CUTS, BREAKS, in this Chapter) and of food poisoning.

One of the main problems with 'staph' is that it produces a toxin (poison) which is *not destroyed by heat*. This also applies to re-heated food. If you have eaten food contaminated by 'staph', the symptoms of severe diarrhoea and vomiting, with stomach pains, will come on within one to six hours. But it usually clears up in a day. For treatment of DIARRHOEA see page 41.

STYES

Treat these in the same way as boils but be very careful to test the heat of the pad before you put it on. The skin of the eyelids is *very* sensitive and delicate and you don't want to scald the patient.

TOOTHACHE

Make sure the family have been to the dentist recently before going on holiday. Treatment from dentists abroad can be very expensive. If a toothache develops and has not disappeared in several hours or gets progressively worse, you should find a doctor as an abscess may have developed. When it reaches a certain stage, the side of the face where the pain is situated will swell up. A doctor will give you the appropriate antibiotics.

10
BITES, STINGS AND RASHES

BITES AND STINGS

'Common' mosquitoes and gnats

Although these are largely harmless, they may be extremely itchy and uncomfortable. An insect repellent such as AUTAN may be used to deter the insects from biting you in the first place.

Once bitten, an antihistamine cream such as ANTHISAN may help to minimise the itching. Also a cream like CALADRYL, which has the same consistency as toothpaste, can be applied to each bite individually.

A nurse I know, who has just returned from an expedition in the jungle, said that if you smeared saliva on the bites this helped to relieve the itching.

There is no other specific treatment. If the bites are bigger and more troublesome than you would normally expect, see a doctor.

It is also a good idea to spray those rooms which you will be using after dark – the bedroom obviously. Two good insecticides are MAFU and VAPONA.

71

Jellyfish

Apart from their nasty sting, they can also give you a considerable shock when you are swimming. Some species are worse than others: the Portuguese Man-O'-War is probably the worst and can be recognised by its bluish purple colour.

Jellyfish seem to vary with the weather and the time of year. If you see one on one day, it is quite likely that there are more around. But the next day there may not be one to be seen. Swimming with a mask and snorkel enables you to see them more easily.

There really is no specific remedy for their sting, but an anti-histamine tablet will help. If some of the barbs are still attached to your skin, rub them off with sand, being careful not to touch them with your bare fingers. Something soothing like CALAMINE lotion will also help. If you develop a fever, then find a doctor.

Scorpions

These are nocturnal and spend the day in dark places, under stones and occasionally in shoes. They will only sting if attacked which does, in their view, include being stepped on by mistake.

For children the effect can be traumatic. They may get a temperature, vomit and have muscular cramps. Apply a heavy, firm pressure to the wound and bandage it, then immobilise the limb as this should delay the movement of the venom.

Call a doctor – a local anaesthetic can help and there is a scorpion anti-venom available for the species found in Mediterranean countries and the Middle East.

Snakes

There are very few people who are not afraid of snakes, but if you remember the following, it should help.

1. Snakes are *not* aggressive: they will do all they can to get out of your way, and bites are very rare.

2. Only 10% of those bitten by the most venomous of snakes actually die. This is partly because the snake rarely injects a full dose of poison.

3. One of the most dangerous aspects of snake bite is the shock. Therefore it is VITAL that you keep the person still, calm, warm and constantly reassured. The more agitated they become, the faster the venom will be carried along the blood stream.

4. The bite of a venomous snake will leave two little holes, or fang marks, whereas the bite of a non-venomous snake will leave two rows of teeth marks and no fangs. However, it is not always that easy to tell so always treat any snake bite as potentially poisonous.

IF BITTEN, you must get the victim to a doctor or hospital immediately but in the meantime, you can do the following:

1. There is much disagreement about the value of making incisions around the bite and trying to suck out the poison. But it seems that unless it is done

immediately, it doesn't help and often results in the area becoming infected as well. So our advice is *not* to try it.

2. Remove any venom off the surface of the skin and wash the bite thoroughly (wipe but don't rub it) with any liquid available.

3. Apply firm pressure over the site of the wound and immobilise the limb until help arrives. Keep the patient as still as possible.

4. If the snake is dead, take it with you for identification. Otherwise, try and memorise what it looked like.

5. You can give ASPIRIN for the pain but preferably *not* alcohol.

6. Remember that however ill the patient seems by the time they are given the anti-venom, the chances of recovery are very good once they have had the injection.

Weever fish

Certainly found in Cornwall and reputedly in Spain, but it seems odd that none are to be found anywhere else – officially anyway. They live below sand or shingle at the sea's edge.

If you step on one, they inject a poison into you and this can be extremely painful. The only known treatment is to immerse your foot in *very* hot water until the pain eases.

Sea Urchins

These are large, black and prickly and are found in the Mediterranean. They stick to the rocks, often at the water's edge. Always check where you are putting your bare feet, or wear shoes. If you tread on one, you must try and remove the barbed spines and keep the area clean and disinfected.

RASHES

There are many causes. The commonest is a *prickly heat rash* with raised red spots which sometimes develop a white head. It most commonly occurs where the skin is moist and tends to rub together, or where the skin is rubbing against clothing all the time. It can be very itchy. Children often develop this kind of rash on their feet.

Treatment:

Keep the area clean and dry and use a medicated powder such as CUTICURA. If the rash is on the feet, then wear cotton and not nylon socks, if socks are necessary at all. Cold showers may keep the area cool and CALAMINE lotion may also soothe the itching.

Other rashes may be caused by *allergies* to various substances or foods (certain medicines, shellfish etc.). These may develop as red wheals on the skin which are usually very itchy. Sometimes vomiting may occur.

These symptoms should disappear within an hour or two BUT if the person becomes worse, or if there are any signs of swelling of the face or tongue (or anywhere else) OR *any* difficulty in breathing, you *must* contact a doctor immediately. The itching may be helped by CALAMINE lotion or cold compresses.

You may have been unlucky enough to have caught a common viral illness (i.e. Chicken Pox) and then to develop the rash when you are abroad. If you are *absolutely sure* that you know what it is – because you have seen other cases of it and you know that it was going round the school or work – then keep the patient at home and make sure that the temperature is kept down (see FEVER page 50).

If there are any other unusual rashes and especially if the person is unwell in any other way, then find a doctor at once.

Nappy Rash

The commonest cause is the effect of wet nappies in contact with the skin. Therefore make sure that nappies are changed frequently and that the baby's bottom is completely clean and dry before another nappy is put on. Baby cream and powder may help to prevent nappy rash. DRAPOLENE, ZINC AND CASTOR OIL or VASOGEN may be used.

Being in a hot country is a good opportunity to expose the baby's bottom to the air as much as possible.

A fungal infection (i.e. thrush) can develop and the baby should be seen by a doctor so that the appropriate cream can be used, such as NYSTAFORM or DAKTARIN.

If the skin has broken, take care not to allow the area to become infected, so take all the precautions as above. You may need a solution such as GENTIAN VIOLET to clear it up.

11
POSSIBLE SEX PROBLEMS

VENEREAL DISEASE (otherwise known as VD, Gonorrhoea, the Clap)

This should not be a problem for the family holiday! However, if you develop a discharge from the penis or the vagina and have a burning sensation when you pass water *and* you have reason to believe that you may have picked this up, then you should contact a doctor, or preferably a specialist clinic, if you can find one.

Precise diagnosis is imperative and you should make every effort to explain everything to the doctor, who will treat whatever you say in confidence. If the infection is not treated it may spread and cause further complications.

Remember that if a woman has had intercourse with a man who has developed symptoms that might indicate VD, she may have the infection without knowing it, as symptoms are not necessarily apparent in a female.

Treatment (until you have seen the doctor):

Ensure strict personal hygiene – wash well and don't use other people's towels. Do not have sexual contact with anyone.

The doctor or clinic will need to know with whom you have had sexual intercourse so that your partner can be protected as well. This may be a difficult and embarrassing business, but if you do not act responsibly about this, you are putting others at great risk of a serious illness.

If you read this BEFORE you have contact with someone you are not sure of, then this may give you cause for thought. But if you do go ahead, then be certain that at least the man wears a protective sheath.

GENITAL HERPES

This is another sexually transmitted disease and can be very painful. It is also very difficult to get rid of. The first infection is usually the worst but it then keeps recurring. It has reached almost epidemic proportions in Europe this year.

Symptoms:

1. The incubation period is 3–7 days and can be accompanied by a general feeling of being unwell, with a possible fever.

2. First visible signs are clusters of little blisters around the genital area, preceded by some local itching. These blisters then form small ulcers which can be very painful or become infected.

3. It may become very painful to urinate.

Treatment:

The blisters/ulcers can last for about 1–2 weeks and then heal of their own accord. The only treatment which seems any good is the application of iodine! Or an ointment called HERPID (which is painful on application and expensive) applied with care. Otherwise, it is best to wait until you get home and can see your own doctor.

12
EMERGENCY FIRST AID

We would like to stress that this is only a holiday guide. For more detailed emergency First Aid measures consult a specialist First Aid book.

CHOKING

Foreign bodies in the lungs are very serious. A person may choke – in other words, the food may go down 'the wrong way', i.e. down the air passages, instead of down the gullet. YOU MUST ACT FAST. If it is a child, try to dislodge the object by tipping him upside down and thumping him on the back.

If it is an adult, give him 3 or 4 hard slaps between the shoulder blades and hopefully they will cough up the object. If the object is not coughed up, or if it has been, but there is still difficulty in breathing, they must go to hospital.

Rules for prevention:

1. NEVER let children play or run with anything in their mouths – particularly sweets, or chewing gum

2. NEVER give peanuts to very young children, since if these go down the

wrong way, they may cause a very severe pneumonia.

CONCUSSION/HEAD INJURY

This results from a blow on the head and can be likened to a shaking-up of the brain, resulting in unconsciousness.

Symptoms:

Unconsciousness, hopefully only for a short time.

The patient feels cold and clammy with a weak pulse as in Fainting/Shock. (see page 84 & 86)

Treatment:

Lie patient on his side with his knees bent and head to one side
Cover with a blanket
Lossen tight clothing
Get a doctor as soon as possible if the patient remains unconscious.
Even when he regains consciousness, it is important that you take him to see a doctor to check that the blow to the head has not caused any other damage.

DROWNING

Prevention is imperative. The following reminders are all obvious and common sense, but we still feel that they are worthwhile outlining:

1. Beware of local swimming conditions, i.e. is the tide going in or out; is the correct beach flag flying indicating that swimming conditions are safe; are other families swimming; are there any known local 'freak' weather conditions; are there jellyfish about, etc.

2. Do not allow children who cannot swim to enter the water without an adult, and keep a very close eye on children who can swim.

3. Do not swim too far out of your depth – which includes floating out on a lilo which can become caught up in strong currents.

4. Do not swim until at least 1½ hours after eating a meal. This can cause cramp. If you get cramp, just tread water until it goes and *don't panic*.

REMEMBER THAT MOST ACCI-DENTS ARE CAUSED BY CARE-LESSNESS

When a person has begun to 'drown' it means that their lungs have become flooded with water and they cannot breathe in air.

Treatment (whilst waiting for medical help to arrive):

Obviously, you have to get the water out of the lungs. QUICKLY tip the person upside down – easy if it is a child – and slap them firmly several times on the back. The idea is to get them to cough so that the water will be expelled from the lungs.

Remove any obstruction in the mouth such as seaweed or false teeth etc. Once the water is removed, then attempt artificial respiration (Kiss of Life).

HEART RESUSCITATION AND ARTIFICIAL RESPIRATION (KISS OF LIFE)

If the person is unconscious for any reason (i.e. drowning) check:

Are they breathing?

Is the heart still going? (Listen with your ear against their chest).

If one of these has stopped, then the other one will soon do so as well. Therefore, heart resuscitation and artificial respiration are VITAL and must be carried out alternately as outlined below.

Lie the person **on their back** on as firm and flat a surface as possible.

Kneel on the right hand side of the patient.

To start the heart:

Thump the chest hard with the edge of your hand towards the bottom of the breast bone and slightly to the patient's left side of the chest. You may get the heart going by doing this without doing anything else.

You can repeat this once or twice.

To keep the heart going:

Place the heel (base of the palm) of your left hand in the centre of the patient's chest and put your right hand on top of your left hand.

Keeping the arms stiff, press down with firm, sharp movements, depressing the chest about 1–2 inches each time (i.e.

a pumping movement).

The rate should be one per second for adults.

For a child, press more gently with *one* hand, and slightly faster.

Kiss of Life:

After 5 heart thumps, the lungs should be expanded as follows:

Firstly, make sure that the mouth is clear of all obstructions and ensure that collars and belts are loose.

Tilt the head well back so that the chin is pointing upwards.

If it is an adult, put your right hand under the chin, then pinch the patient's nostrils shut with your other hand.

Take a deep breath.

Then place your mouth directly over the patient's so that no air can escape.

Blow *hard* into the patient's mouth until you see his chest rise. Then stop and allow the air to be exhaled naturally from the lungs.

If it is a child do exactly the same thing but place your mouth over his *mouth and nose*.

After you have blown into the patient's mouth **once**, give him another 5 of the heart thumps.

Continue to repeat this sequence, until the patient starts to breathe again, or until medical help arrives.

FAINTING

There are many causes but what happens is that the blood pressure drops, and if it drops too low, you lose consciousness.

Symptoms:

The patient feels light-headed and weak.

Vision becomes blurred and voices nearby seem far away.

He may feel dizzy and may vomit.

The observer will notice that the patient has become pale, particularly around the lips, and that he seems a bit vacant. The skin may become clammy and the pulse may be weak.

Treatment:

If the patient is relatively well otherwise, it may be enough to sit him on a chair with his head between his knees. He should recover quickly and should then be given a drink with sugar in it, preferably a warm one.

If the patient is actually about to lose consciousness or has already done so, THEN;

Lie him on the ground FAST on his back, with his head turned to one side, and raise his legs in the air.

Loosen tight clothing anywhere on the body (i.e. collars and belts).

Cover him with a blanket but DON'T give him a hot water bottle.

Stay with him and reassure him as he might be frightened.

A simple faint should improve quickly, with the patient coming round almost immediately, but he should stay lying down until he feels well and then be given warm sweet drinks.

If a fit young person faints, and there is an obvious reason for it, then there should be nothing to worry about. If an elderly person faints, then it is important to get medical attention, particularly if he does not come round quickly.

SHOCK

This can result from many different causes, but it is essentially a very severe form of fainting, as described above. The commonest cause is when someone has been involved in an accident and/or has broken a limb and/or is bleeding.

Get someone to call a doctor IMMEDIATELY.

Lie the patient down and DO NOT move him.

Try to stop the bleeding with firm pressure over the wound (if there are any people standing around, they will tell you not to touch the patient, but to stand by and watch a patient bleeding would be irresponsible). If his nose is bleeding, pinch his nostrils together.

I was once at the scene of an accident when a man had been run over by a car. There was blood everywhere. The other bystanders kept saying 'don't touch him', but on closer examination, I realised that the blood was coming from his nose. He had already lost a lot of blood, and if I *had* left him to bleed, he would have lost a lot more. By pinching his nostrils together I was able to stop the bleeding, although *at no time* did I move him in any way.

Otherwise, do the commonsense thing, as in FAINTING (page 84) but DO NOT give him anything to eat or drink even if he is fully conscious, as he may need an anaesthetic.

13
MISCELLANEOUS

ANTIBIOTICS

This subject seems to cause a lot of controversy and confusion. But there are several useful guidelines to remember:

1. They should never be taken unless prescribed by a doctor. You may take the wrong one OR far more seriously, you may mask the symptoms of a serious illness OR the organism may become resistant to the antibiotic. If you suffer from chronic problems such as tonsillitis, cystitis or chest infections, then your doctor may be willing to give you some appropriate medicine to take with you just to be on the safe side. But even then do not take them until you get appropriate symptoms and/or only if you are sure of what you are treating.

2. They do not kill viruses, therefore they are not used for common coughs and colds.

3. They should not be given for diarrhoea unless specifically indicated.

4. They should be taken for a COMPLETE course. Do NOT just stop when you think you are better.

5. If, after taking them, you develop a skin rash or become itchy, then you must stop taking them immediately. Tell your doctor when you get home and *never* take that particular one again except on medical advice. Obviously, if you develop more serious allergic symptoms, such as swelling of the face or difficulty in breathing, then you must find a doctor *immediately*.

CHEST PAIN

If a person complains of any sort of unexplained pain in the chest they should be seen by a doctor.

CONSTIPATION

Everybody has different bowel habits. Some go once a day, some every few days. Constipation is when *your* personal routine is prolonged by several days or when you are passing very hard stools. If you eat the correct food i.e. vegetables, bran, fruit and enough fluids such as orange juice, then this should not be a problem and you should not have to resort to medicine. Always try the natural method first, especially drinking more fluids.

When the natural methods have failed, try any of the following: MILPAR: MILK OF MAGNESIA (a gentle laxative especially good for children, although they don't usually like taking it!) DULCOLAX: SENOKOT.

If a child becomes constipated but is otherwise *completely* well, and the natural methods have not worked, then try one of the medicines mentioned, taking care to give the smaller doses recommended. If the child is unwell in any other way, i.e. vomiting or has abdominal pain, then get a doctor.

CYSTITIS (sometimes called the Honeymoon disease)

This is usually a feminine problem and is often connected with sexual intercourse. The symptoms are a burning sensation when you urinate, cloudy urine which may have a bad smell, and sometimes may have blood in it – and abdominal pain over the lower part of the tummy.

Until you can get to a doctor, drink plenty of fluids such as Barley Water. Don't drink alcohol or eat spicy foods. Hot baths, a hot water bottle and pain killers will help ease the pain. The doctor will put you on a course of antibiotics.

If you get recurrent cystitis, remember to ask your doctor for a supply of antibiotics before you go away. If you get a bout of it when you are abroad, tell your doctor when you get home. This is particularly important in the case of a man since there may be serious underlying problems.

EARACHE

If a child develops earache, especially if he looks flushed and unwell, then he probably has an infection in a part of the ear that you cannot see (middle ear). You must find a doctor who will give the child an appropriate antibiotic. In the meantime, give PARACETAMOL to lower the temperature and ease the pain. Make sure an ear infection is cleared up before flying.

Remember that a very young child may be unable to localise the pain – but if he is unwell with a fever for no obvious reason, he will have to see a doctor anyway.

Some children develop ear infections when they have a cold. If fluid or pus comes out of the ear, then find a doctor even if the pain by this time has gone.

Do not allow a child in these circumstances to swim.

A sharp cold wind can also cause earache but this is only temporary.

Wax in the ear does not usually cause pain. If it does, *warm* olive oil can be poured into the ear and kept there with the head turned to one side to loosen the wax. CERUMOL eardrops can also be used.

If there is a pain in the ear, a discharge (other than wax) or a temperature, then a doctor must be found.

Beware, also, of foreign bodies in the ear (see FOREIGN BODIES page 66)

HEADACHES

You may be prone to getting these and so will have taken the appropriate pain-relief medicine with you. But if the headache is more severe than normal and if there are no obvious reasons why, (too much sun for example) then find a doctor.

With children any headache should be treated with care as it is unusual for them to have them. Remember that young children are often unable to localise the pain and this makes it more difficult.

If the headache is accompanied by vomiting or fever OR spots OR a sensitivity to the light OR if the child is otherwise unwell, then *get a doctor*. The chances are that the headache will disappear quickly and that the child will feel fine, BUT it may be a sign of MENINGITIS. If a child lies with its head and neck bent back or is unable to sit up and kiss its bent knees, *GET A DOCTOR AT ONCE or, preferably get to a hospital first. Do not* give a child with these symptoms antibiotics.

SCABIES

This can be caught anywhere, but personal hygiene will certainly help you prevent catching it. It is caused by a mite which invades the skin, leaving little burrows which result in a very itchy rash, especially on the wrists, between the toes and fingers and in the genital area. CALAMINE can help but try and wait until you get home where it can be dealt with effectively.

VAGINAL DISCHARGE (Thrush)

This is normally a white discharge which causes itching in the vulval area, and is caused by the yeast called Candida (Thrush). If you can put up with the discomfort, and you are only on a 2–3 week holiday, it may be simpler to consult your doctor when you get home, who will take a swab and prescribe the correct treatment.

14
VISITING AUSTRALIA AND NEW ZEALAND

The Australian medical services are just as modern and good as those here and in the United States. Their emergency services are excellent and should you have a health problem of any kind, you will be looked after extremely efficiently and well.

There are none of the following illnesses: Cholera, Typhoid, Malaria, Rabies, Brucellosis. But there are a few 'dangers' which are as follows:

SPIDERS

There are two types of spider which can kill. They are:
   Red back spider
   Funnel web spider

Red Back Spider

This is fat and round, the size of a pea, with a dark blackish brown body with a red or orange stripe down its back. It is often found in gardens and under rubbish. Only the female bites.

Symptoms of bite:

Pain initially round bite and then becoming general
Dizziness, nausea and possibly vomiting
Faintness and muscular weakness
You can sweat profusely
Swelling around the bite
Muscular spasm

Treatment:

Get medical help *immediately*, but in the meantime:

Wipe the bite clean and if you have any ice or cold water handy, put on a cold compress (made of a combination of ice cubes and water) while you are getting the bandage ready.

Put on a crêpe bandage (or similar) on the limb on the side of the bite nearest to the heart and bandage firmly.

It is important to keep the limb still so put on some sort of splint – anything to keep the limb rigid.

Whatever you do, keep the patient calm and reassured. Don't leave him alone if you can help it. Don't give him alcohol.

Someone should try and catch the spider so that it can be taken, dead or alive, to the hospital.

Anti-venom serum is available for this spider.

Funnel Web Spider

Large and black with a body about 3cm. long. They frequent moist dark areas (such as dustbin sheds) or damp caves and

crevices. They are found in Sydney mainly
and on the Eastern coast of New South
Wales.

Symptoms of the bite:

The bite hurts to start with but there is
little local reaction
It is difficult to breathe and the pulse is
rapid
There is a numbness; your muscles feel
weak
You sweat profusely
Copious salivary and bronchial secretions
Spasm of the larynx

Treatment:

see Red Back spider (page 92).

There are lots of other big, hairy and
horrid looking spiders in Australia, but
they are perfectly harmless. As being
bitten by anything is a shock, it is very
important to reassure and calm the person
down. The more agitated he becomes, the
faster the venom moves through the blood-
stream.

SNAKES

There are lots of venomous snakes in
Australia, so if you are bitten, treat it as a
potentially venomous bite. Follow the same
procedure as for spiders – bandage firmly
with a crêpe bandage and get medical help
fast. For more general information on
snake bites, see BITES, STINGS, ETC.
(page 71).

BLUE BOTTLES

These are little creatures like jellyfish which can sting you when you are swimming. They are a nuisance in the summer season and especially in the Queensland area.

If you have any methylated spirits with you, rub a little on and take an antihistamine tablet.

STONE FISH

These are found in coral reef areas and are difficult to see because they do look like stones. Their sting is very dangerous and you must get medical help *IMMEDIATELY*.

Symptoms:

The area of the sting throbs, stings, turns blue and then red

Bleeding may be heavy and the limb becomes swollen

Sweating is followed by a collapse in the circulation system

Breathing becomes difficult and the muscles can become paralysed.

Treatment (whilst medical help is being found):

Check to see if the person is breathing. If not, give KISS OF LIFE (see page 84).

Check the pulse and if it is very slow or has stopped, you will have to pump the heart (see page 82).

When these emergencies have been dealt with, clean the wound with water.

Remove any foreign bodies from the

wound and immerse the affected part in hot water – as hot as can be tolerated as this may neutralise the toxin.

Note: There is an anti-venom for stone fish.

A FINAL WORD

We hope that the contents of this book have not put you off going abroad on holiday. It is very unlikely that you will have any major problems, but you may encounter some minor ones, such as diarrhoea. Our main hope is that all this information will give you the confidence to deal with most of the problems yourself, and to know when you MUST find medical help.

On the following page is an emergency vocabulary – just the key words that may be necessary.

Dutch and the Scandinavian languages have not been included as in these countries English is almost universally spoken, and if not English, then German is fully understood.

So far as the Middle East is concerned, we felt it too difficult to give a crash course in the various Arabic, and Hebrew tongues. In any case, a European language, either English or French is usually understood in these areas.

Obviously you should take the relevant phrase book with you where you will also have help with phonetic pronunciation.

ENGLISH	FRENCH	GERMAN	SPANISH	ITALIAN	GREEK	TURKISH
DOCTOR	docteur	doktor	doctor	dottore	iatros	doktor
HOSPITAL	hôpital	krankenhaus	hospital	ospedale	nosokomion	hastane
PAIN: STOMACH	mal au ventre	schmerzen:–bauch	dolor de abdomen	male di stomacho	pono:–stomach	karinarisi basarisa
PAIN: HEAD	mal de tête	schmerzen:–kopf	dolor de cabeza	male di testa	pono:–kefalos	
DIARRHOEA	diarrhée	durchfall	diarrea	diarrea	diarrea	idirar
UNCONSCIOUS	inconscient	besinnungslos	inconsciente	inconscio	anaisthitos	baygin
ACCIDENT	accident	unfall	accidente	incidente	dystychima	kaza
BROKEN BONE	os cassé	knocken-bruch	hueso roto	osso rotto	spasmeno	kenik
CONVULSION	convulsion	anfall	convulsion	convulsione	jokokalo epilepsia	kirionis ihtilác
FEVER	fièvre	fieber	fiebre	febre	piretos	humma
BLOOD	sang	blut	sangre	sangue	aima	tan
BABY	bébé	kindchen	bebe	bimbo	moro	bebek

INDEX

A

B

C

NOTES

NOTES